Women and psychosis

An information guide

Pamela Blake, MSW, RSW
April A. Collins, MSW, RSW
Mary V. Seeman, MD
Revised by Mary V. Seeman, MD

camh
Centre for Addiction and Mental Health

A Pan American Health Organization /
World Health Organization Collaborating Centre

Library and Archives Canada Cataloguing in Publication

Blake, Pamela, 1954-, author
    Women and psychosis : an information guide : a guide for women and their families / Pamela Blake, MSW, RSW, April A. Collins, MSW, RSW, Mary V. Seeman, MD. -- Revised edition / revised by Mary V. Seeman, MD

"A Pan American Health Organization/World Health Organization Collaborating Centre."
Includes bibliographical references.
Issued in print and electronic formats.
ISBN 978-1-77052-635-8 (paperback).--ISBN 978-1-77052-636-5 (pdf).--
ISBN 978-1-77052-637-2 (html).--ISBN 978-1-77052-638-9 (epub).--
ISBN 978-1-77114-237-3 (kindle)

        1. Women--Mental health. 2. Psychoses. 3. Mentally ill women--
Family relationships. I. Collins, April, author II. Seeman, M. V.
(Mary Violette), 1935-, author III. Centre for Addiction and Mental
Health, issuing body IV. Title.

RC512.B52 2015   616.890082   C2015-906423-6
                                                C2015-906424-4

Printed in Canada

This publication may be available in other formats. For information about alternative formats or other CAMH publications, or to place an order, please contact Sales and Distribution:
Toll-free: 1 800 661-1111
Toronto: 416 595-6059
E-mail: publications@camh.ca
Online store: http://store.camh.ca
Website: www.camh.ca

Disponible en français sous le titre
La psychose chez les femmes : Guide à l'intention des femmes et de leurs familles

This guide was produced by CAMH Education.

3973m / 02-2016 / PM119

Contents

Acknowledgments

We owe special thanks to the many clients, their families and the staff of the following programs and organizations who reviewed an earlier version of this information guide or assisted with the review process:

Best Practices Services, Whitby Mental Health Centre, Whitby, Ontario

Canadian Mental Health Association, Cornwall, Ontario

Can-Voice, London, Ontario

Community Programs, Centre for Addiction and Mental Health, London, Toronto, Oshawa and Cornwall, Ontario

Family Advisory Group, Centre for Addiction and Mental Health, Toronto, Ontario

Schizophrenia and Continuing Care Program, Centre for Addiction and Mental Health, Toronto, Ontario

Skills Training Treatment and Education Place (STEP), Whitby Mental Health Centre, Whitby, Ontario

Introduction

This guide is for women who are recovering from a psychotic episode. The information will also be useful for their families.

Psychotic illness affects women and men in somewhat different ways. In women, schizophrenia—the most common form of psychotic illness—usually starts later in life than it does in men, and progresses at a different pace. This means that treatment for women may not be the same as it is for men. Treatment outcomes also differ between men and women. Textbooks often talk about psychosis, its treatment and its outcomes as if gender differences were unimportant. This guide, on the other hand, focuses on the specific issues that women and their families face during recovery from psychosis.

1 About psychosis

What is psychosis?

The word psychosis is used to describe conditions that affect the mind, in which people have trouble distinguishing between what is real and what is not.

Approximately three out of 100 people will experience a period of psychosis in their lifetime. Psychosis affects men and women equally and occurs across all cultures and socioeconomic groups.

Experiencing psychosis is frightening, confusing and distressing to most people. It is also confusing to those who witness someone struggling with psychotic thoughts, which may lead to misconceptions about what is happening that further add to the person's distress.

What causes psychosis?

Many factors can contribute to psychosis, including high fever, drug use, starvation, hormonal problems, neurological illness such as epilepsy, immune reactions and hereditary or early life factors.

Often the cause is unknown, and the illness appears to come "out of the blue."

During a period of psychosis, a woman may come to believe things that are not true. These false beliefs are called delusions. She may believe, for instance, that her partner is cheating on her. She may see meanings in her partner's actions, gestures and tone of voice that are based on her worst fears, not on reality. A woman having a psychotic episode may hear a voice in her head confirming her fears, which she takes as proof that her beliefs are true. It is difficult to change such fixed beliefs, even if there is evidence that contradicts them.

Sometimes delusions stem from a change in mood. For example, if a woman is very depressed, she may feel unlovable; this may lead her to falsely believe that she is being abandoned, discriminated against or attacked.

It is always difficult to determine the precise underlying causes of psychotic symptoms. And symptoms change over time, making it harder to understand their causes. There is no objective test for psychosis. The diagnosis is based on:
· what the woman (and her family) reports
· the duration of symptoms
· how much the symptoms interfere with everyday functioning.

Do women and men experience psychosis differently?

Women and men are equally likely to develop psychosis. However, there are differences in the way the illness may affect women and men.

While psychosis related to drug use is more common in men than in women, psychosis associated with mood changes or thyroid disease is more common in women.

Typically, women's delusions focus on relationships; the false belief that a partner is cheating is a common delusion in women experiencing psychosis. Men's delusions generally involve more abstract concerns.

Women tend to have fewer "negative" symptoms of schizophrenia (that is, a loss or reduction of normal functioning) than men. These negative symptoms include loss of pleasure, motivation or social interaction. Women also have fewer cognitive symptoms of schizophrenia, such as trouble with attention, reasoning and memory, than men do.

On the other hand, mood-related symptoms of schizophrenia, especially symptoms of depression such as crying easily, guilt and loss of hope, are more common in women. Psychotic illness usually affects men for the first time in their late teens and women for the first time in their twenties. The later onset gives women the advantage of having more schooling behind them when they first become ill. Women also have more relationship and work experience by that time, which helps with recovery.

Women are thought to respond better to treatments for psychosis than men do. For instance, women seem to do well with relatively low doses of antipsychotic medication. In general, women tend to be more open to talking about their experiences and, therefore, also do better than men with psychosocial treatments such as psychotherapy. This is good news for women.

However, women go through times when the risk of a recurrence of psychosis is high. These include premenstrual, childbirth and postpartum periods, and menopause. This suggests that women's hormones may affect their vulnerability to psychosis. Other risk factors include poverty, immigration, substance use, domestic abuse, sexual exploitation and single parenthood. In addition, thyroid problems and steroid drugs (used for arthritis and for allergies) are greater risk factors for women than for men.

Forms of Psychosis

SCHIZOPHRENIA

Schizophrenia is characterized by three clusters of symptoms.

The first cluster is positive symptoms—those that *add to or distort* the person's normal functioning. Positive symptoms include delusions (fixed beliefs not based in fact) and hallucinations (hearing, seeing, tasting, smelling or feeling something that isn't actually there).

The second cluster is negative symptoms—loss or distortion of normal functioning. Negative symptoms include loss of pleasure, motivation and initiative; feeling apathetic; showing little emotion and avoiding social contact.

The third cluster is cognitive symptoms, such as impairment of memory and of reasoning and calculating abilities.

For a diagnosis of schizophrenia to be made, these three clusters of symptoms must have lasted for at least six months, and must have interfered with the person's ability to function.

Schizophrenia is a long-lasting illness. Remissions (periods when a person has no symptoms) occur, but the person needs to continue treatment even during a remission in order to prevent relapse (the return of symptoms).

SCHIZOPHRENIFORM DISORDER

This term is used for symptoms of schizophrenia that have not yet lasted for six months. Schizophreniform disorder may disappear on its own or may develop into a longer-lasting illness.

BIPOLAR DISORDER

Bipolar disorder is a mood illness that alternates between periods of depression and periods of elevated mood (mania). When psychotic symptoms arise, they often reflect the person's mood. For example, people who are depressed may hear voices that put them down. People who are experiencing elevated mood may believe they are special and are capable of doing amazing things.

SCHIZOAFFECTIVE DISORDER

During this type of psychosis, a person experiences symptoms of both schizophrenia and mood disturbance. The two kinds of symptoms may appear at the same time or may alternate.

DEPRESSION WITH PSYCHOTIC FEATURES

Sometimes a person will experience a severe depression with symptoms of psychosis, without the mania associated with bipolar disorder. This type of depression is referred to as a psychotic depression or depression with psychotic features.

DRUG-INDUCED PSYCHOSIS

The use of drugs such as marijuana, cocaine, ecstasy, ketamine, LSD, amphetamines and alcohol can sometimes trigger psychotic symptoms. Once the effects of the drugs wear off, the symptoms of psychosis will usually go away. If they do not go away, the drug use may have triggered a longer-lasting illness.

BRIEF PSYCHOTIC DISORDER

Sometimes symptoms of psychosis come on suddenly and, in some cases, are triggered by a major stress in the person's life, such as a death in the family. This type of psychosis lasts less than a month, and is more common in women than in men.

DELUSIONAL DISORDER

A delusional disorder is a long-lasting illness in which delusions (usually one elaborate delusion) are prominent, but in which there are no hallucinations. An example of an elaborate delusion is a person believing that a song she wrote has been stolen by a popular band, and that this band has made millions of dollars from the song. The person devotes her life to "setting the record straight" and, in so doing, neglects everything else in her life. A delusional disorder may not prevent normal functioning in some areas of life, but it strains relationships.

Posttraumatic Stress Disorder (PTSD)

This term usually refers to non-psychotic symptoms that follow a traumatic experience such as a violent assault, but psychotic symptoms may also sometimes arise. The affected person relives the event, is preoccupied with it, avoids situations associated with it and may have flashbacks (visual and auditory recollections of the event) that are difficult to distinguish from the hallucinations of a psychotic illness. More women than men develop PTSD symptoms when exposed to a traumatic event.

Diagnosis

It may be difficult to make a diagnosis in the early stages of psychosis. Often patterns of symptoms must be assessed over many months, and determining a diagnosis may take some time. To help your doctor make an accurate diagnosis, it is important to be as thorough as possible when telling him or her what you are experiencing. Let your doctor know what you have been thinking and feeling. If you have been using alcohol or other drugs, tell your doctor how much and how recently. If you have been traumatized, either as a child or as an adult, tell your doctor. You also need to discuss any family history of mental health problems.

It may be distressing or confusing to talk to a health care professional, especially when you are not feeling well. The symptoms of illness may interfere with your ability to express yourself. Your doctor or other members of your health care team may ask for your consent to speak to your family or close friends. Family and friends can give information about what they have observed that may help with the diagnosis.

The more information your doctor has, the more likely he or she is to make the most accurate diagnosis and recommend the most effective treatment.

2 Recovering from psychosis

What is recovery?

Recovery from psychosis does not necessarily mean losing all symptoms or being able to move forward without treatment. It means returning to normal activities and functioning, gaining a sense of control over one's life, and recovering hope and faith in the future.

Issues for today's women

In our society, poverty, domestic abuse and childhood sexual abuse are experienced more often by women than by men. Other life pressures may include relative lack of autonomy and cultural expectations to be slim, and to be a perfect mother and a family caretaker, all while holding down a full-time job. In some households, these issues loom very large. In addition, immigrant and refugee women may face discrimination, exploitation, isolation and language barriers. It is suspected that such pressures contribute to the expression of psychosis and affect the speed of recovery.

Common questions about recovering from psychosis

SINCE BECOMING ILL, I'M NOT FEELING VERY GOOD ABOUT MYSELF. IS THIS NORMAL?

The experience of psychosis is a life crisis. It is a trauma that may, in itself, lead to a posttraumatic stress reaction. It is hard to know what to expect of the future after an episode of psychosis.

In addition, negative stereotypes (stigma) about people with mental illness still exist in many communities. This stigma has a negative impact on people living with psychosis. If you are not feeling good about yourself, ask yourself whether this is due to stigma, depression, fear about the future or lingering symptoms of the illness.

It may help to sort out your feelings if you discuss them with a trusted family member, friend or therapist. Talking things over will help you rebuild confidence and decide on the next steps in recovery. Some women find it useful to attend a support group for women who have had similar experiences.

WHAT CAN I DO TO RECOVER FROM MY ILLNESS?

As you try to regain control over your life, it is important to work closely with your doctor and other health care providers. Together, you can explore the personal risk factors that may have contributed to the illness. It is important to learn as much as possible about what may have caused the episode, so that similar situations can be avoided in the future. Therapists usually recommend plenty of sleep, exercise, a nutritious diet, a social support network, positive family connections, meaningful work and structured days. Often, regular appointments with a mental health worker and low-dose medications are needed to keep psychosis at bay.

Recovery after psychosis does not happen quickly or easily. It usually takes time and occurs in gradual steps.

Questions about medications

WHAT MEDICATIONS ARE USED TO TREAT PSYCHOSIS?

Antipsychotic medications are considered to be the foundation of treatment for psychosis. To prevent relapse, medication is usually continued after the psychosis is over. Newer antipsychotic medications are always being developed.

Antipsychotic medications that are currently commonly used in Canada include olanzapine (Zyprexa), risperidone (Risperdal), quetiapine (Seroquel), clozapine (Clozaril) and ziprasidone (Zeldox). Some are available in injectable, long-acting preparations.

Other medications may also be prescribed for problems that sometimes accompany psychosis or that are side-effects of antipsychotic medications. These problems may include missed menstrual periods, stiff muscles, sleep problems, depression, anxiety, weight gain, diabetes or mood swings.

DO WOMEN RESPOND DIFFERENTLY TO MEDICATIONS THAN MEN DO?

Women usually need lower doses of medications than men do both in acute phases of illness and in maintenance phases (when symptoms are under control). However, this may not be true after menopause. Women may need lower doses because they absorb and metabolize drugs differently than men do. Medication dose is also affected by diet, weight, genetics, smoking, drinking alcohol, or using other prescription or street drugs. Antipsychotic medications tend to accumulate in fat cells of the body, and so last longer in women's bodies because women, on average, have more fatty tissue than men have.

DO WOMEN EXPERIENCE ANY SIDE-EFFECTS?

All medications may have some unwanted side-effects. In most cases, side-effects are not serious, and they often respond to treatment or disappear as therapy continues. You may experience some side-effects before you notice the benefits of your medication. This is a sign that the drug is being absorbed into the body and is beginning to work. It is unwise to stop your medication without checking with your doctor first.

Side-effects vary with the dose and type of medication. Some women have almost no side-effects, or very mild ones. Others have side-effects that are more severe and troubling. Each person's responses are unique. Be sure to tell your doctor about any side-effects you experience.

Most drugs used in psychiatry decrease metabolism and so cause weight gain. This is a serious problem for most women and requires careful attention to diet and exercise. It contributes to a higher risk of diabetes and cardiovascular disease. Let your doctor know if there is diabetes or cardiovascular disease in your family, and be sure to have regular medical checks.

Menstruation and reproduction

Many drugs used in psychiatry block transmission of the neuro-chemical dopamine, which in turn increases the secretion of the hormone prolactin. This process may interfere with menstrual periods. Importantly, it does *not* signify either pregnancy or meno-pause. Let your doctor know if there is a change in your menstrual cycle. If at all possible, your doctor will adjust your medications so that menstruation is not interrupted. Despite the absence of periods, pregnancy is still possible, so be sure to continue the use of contra-ception unless you are hoping for children. It is important to discuss contraceptive issues with your doctor or mental health worker.

The rise in prolactin can cause other side-effects, such as breast tenderness or swelling and, sometimes, milk flowing from the breasts. Some women find these side-effects very uncomfortable. Another side-effect can be vaginal dryness. Some women also feel less interested in sex than usual or may be unable to reach orgasm. It is important to discuss sexual side-effects with your health care provider.

Drowsiness and passivity

Medications may also cause drowsiness or feelings of passivity. Feeling passive means that, instead of standing up for yourself, it is easier to just "go along." In domestic situations, women may find themselves taken advantage of because their medications make them passive. In some work, driving or caretaking situations, the sedative effect can be very dangerous and needs to be discussed with your doctor. There are usually simple ways to deal with it.

Tardive dyskinesia

Some drugs used for psychosis can cause involuntary movements (tardive dyskinesia, or TD) after some time, especially in older people. You may not notice these movements, but your doctor needs to screen for them.

Other side-effects

Other side-effects can include constipation, muscle stiffness, restlessness, anxiety, insomnia, drooling or nightmares. Rarely, epileptic-like seizures may occur.

HOW LONG WILL I NEED TO TAKE MEDICATION?

There is no single answer to this question: it depends on the course of illness, which is unpredictable. Some women continue to take a low dose of medication throughout their life to prevent recurrence of psychotic illness. Some find that the beginning of menopause makes symptoms temporarily worse, and they need higher doses at that time. Discuss all medication concerns with your doctor.

IS IT OK TO DRINK ALCOHOL WHEN I'M TAKING MEDICATION?

The occasional glass of wine or beer should not trouble most people. However, drinking a lot can lead to a recurrence of psychosis. Specialized counselling exists for women who have problems with alcohol or other drug use.

WHAT ABOUT THE EFFECT OF TAKING OTHER DRUGS?

It is very clear that using street drugs worsens psychotic symptoms. Even if you are free of symptoms, drug use can cause symptoms to return, which may require hospitalization.

Over-the-counter and prescription medications, herbal remedies, caffeine and tobacco may also interact with antipsychotic medication. Caffeine raises the blood level of some antipsychotics.

Smoking may affect how your body processes your medication. Many smokers need to take larger doses of some medications. You should talk to your doctor or pharmacist about drug interactions.

DO BIRTH CONTROL PILLS AFFECT MY MEDICATION?

Birth control pills, or oral contraceptives, contain the female hormones estradiol and progesterone. These hormones can inhibit liver enzymes that process your prescribed drugs. When this happens, more of the drug goes into your bloodstream. As a result, the blood levels of antipsychotic drugs may rise and unwanted side-effects can occur. It is best to consult your doctor about how birth control pills and some antipsychotic drugs might interact.

WHAT OTHER TYPES OF BIRTH CONTROL COULD I CONSIDER?

Some women prefer barrier methods, such as the male or female condom or a diaphragm. Insisting that all male partners wear condoms during sexual intercourse is probably best. Condoms not only minimize the risk of unwanted pregnancy, but also help stop viruses, such as HIV, or other infections from spreading. You may find it hard to ensure that a male partner wears a condom at all times. If so, it is best to consult your doctor about what else is available. New products are being developed.

You may want to check the availability of morning-after pills, and to ask your doctor whether they would be a good option for you. You may find it useful to attend sex education classes, where you can learn about the large choice of contraceptives in everyday use. You can also learn how to say "no" to unwanted sexual advances. It is important to protect yourself against abuse and harassment.

CAN ANTIPSYCHOTIC MEDICATIONS TAKE NUTRIENTS AWAY FROM MY BODY?

Some prescription medications may affect how the body absorbs and processes vitamins and minerals. More needs to be learned about this topic. It is useful to have your doctor take a blood test periodically to check your levels of folates and vitamin B. You may also wish to speak to a nutritionist or pharmacist.

CAN I TAKE MEDICATIONS DURING PREGNANCY?

The first trimester (three months) of pregnancy is a crucial time for making choices. Women must decide whether to continue with the pregnancy and the drug regimen.

It is generally best to avoid all medications during pregnancy and breastfeeding. This is not always possible, however, and a mother's first obligation to her fetus and infant is to stay as healthy as possible. Most of the drugs discussed in this book are not associated with fetal abnormalities if taken during pregnancy, but they may have other side-effects for pregnant women and for newborns. Pregnancy is a time to stay in very close touch with your doctor. Medications may need to be changed or their doses adjusted.

The Motherisk program at the Hospital for Sick Children, in Toronto, is an international resource for information on using medications during pregnancy. Consulting with the Motherisk program is highly recommended (tel.: 416 813-6780; website: www.motherisk.org).

Pregnancy should be carefully planned. Doctors recommend that women start taking a folate supplement before pregnancy begins to prevent neural tube defects. These defects can occur for any pregnant woman, but may be more common among women taking medications or those who are overweight. Because of hormonal changes and psychological stresses, the postpartum period can be a very vulnerable time in which psychotic symptoms may recur for some women.

CAN I TAKE MEDICATIONS WHILE BREASTFEEDING?

Breastfeeding is important for the mother-baby bond and the health of the baby. There are breastfeeding schedules that minimize the amount of a medication that is transmitted to a breastfeeding infant.

ARE HERBAL REMEDIES EFFECTIVE?

To date, there is not enough evidence to support using herbal medicines to treat psychosis. Some herbal remedies may actually provoke psychiatric symptoms. More research is needed in this area. Because of potential drug interactions, it is important to inform your doctor if you take any herbal remedies.

Questions about other treatments

Non-drug treatments are especially important to women because they can be used safely during pregnancy.

WHAT OTHER TREATMENTS ARE AVAILABLE, BESIDES MEDICATION?

· Psychoeducation: Learning about your illness and its treatment is crucial. This will help you to make informed treatment decisions, and to stay as healthy as possible.
· Rehabilitation: A rehabilitation program can help you regain

confidence and learn new skills.

· Psychotherapy: Therapy or counselling can help you cope with
illness. Cognitive therapy, which focuses on the links between
thoughts, feelings and actions, can teach you how to cope with
specific symptoms. Individual or group, marital and family counselling are all available. Support for the family is also important.
Parents, siblings, partners and children are all deeply affected
by a relative's psychosis. They need to learn how to support their
family member and how to cope with troubling symptoms. They
also need the chance to talk about their concerns.

IS SHOCK TREATMENT EVER USED FOR PSYCHOSIS?

Shock treatment, or electroconvulsive therapy (ECT), is sometimes
advised for people with psychosis who do not respond to medication. Patients are given muscle relaxants and a general anesthetic
before a mild electrical current is applied to one side of the brain.
Current ECT treatments cause little memory loss compared with
the older forms. The amount of memory loss depends on the num-
ber of consecutive treatments, the time between treatments, and
the person's unique response.

WHAT IS TMS?

Transcranial magnetic stimulation (TMS) is a new form of treatment that applies magnetic waves to the brain. TMS is helpful for
specific symptoms, such as hallucinations.

3 How psychosis affects family and friends

How will my illness affect my family?

This is a difficult period for the family. A family member may have had to bring you to hospital against your will because he or she was afraid for your safety. The psychosis may have been as frightening for the family as for you. It is very common for families to feel unsettled and distressed at this time. These feelings may last for the first weeks, and sometimes months, after the illness begins.

Families often act in an overprotective way, because they want to shield you from further pain. At times, it may feel as if they are taking over and deciding everything for you. This often stirs up negative feelings. It can be especially hard if you are used to living independently.

Working with family members on how to manage the illness is very challenging. It often takes a lot of time and negotiation for family members to find the right balance between being protective and respecting your independence. Speak with your doctor and other health care providers about how to sort out independence issues with your family.

How will my illness affect my friends?

Friends are often very loyal, but you may be embarrassed at how
you behaved while you were ill and so may feel like isolating
yourself. Try as much as possible to renew friendships and not
to let illness affect your relationships. Some friends will be more
understanding than others. Some friends may drift away. On the
other hand, you may make new friendships with people who have
experienced and overcome similar difficulties.

RESUMING CONTACT

You might feel shy about contacting your friends if you haven't
seen them for a while. You may be afraid they'll reject you if they
learn that you've been ill. It's up to you to decide what to tell your
friends about your illness and treatment.

You may benefit from talking with a counsellor about questions
such as: Who would you like to tell about your illness? How much
do you want to tell your friends? How are they likely to react? How
will you feel as a result?

FEELING PRESSURE TO CONFORM

After a psychotic episode, you may feel that you have changed
and have little in common with your old friends. You have had an
experience that your friends have not had. Feeling different may
also come from changing parts of your past lifestyle. For example,
if you previously used street drugs or drank alcohol, and you no
longer do so, you may feel pressured to rejoin your friends in
these activities. This may be tempting if you want to fit in and
feel "normal." Also, because they may not know much about the

illness or medication, friends might urge you to stop taking your pills. This is bad advice. Always discuss any medication concerns with your doctor or counsellor.

4 Getting back on track

Your illness may have interrupted your studies or work life. If so, it may be very upsetting to see your friends moving ahead in their lives. Hard as it may be, you are better off returning to your activities slowly. Jumping back into work or school can interfere with recovery. After all, you wouldn't run a marathon the day after having a cast removed from a mended broken leg. Taking small steps at first will increase your chances of reaching your goals.

Returning to work or school

You need to decide with your doctor or counsellor what kinds of activities to do and how much. Some of the following factors may affect your choice.

WHAT ARE YOUR VALUES?

How important is it to you to go to school or work right now? Are there other activities that might satisfy you, such as hobbies or volunteer work?

HOW WELL DO YOU FEEL?

Even when psychotic symptoms are well controlled, women may struggle with other issues. They may note changes in how they remember and concentrate. Or they may feel a change in their energy level. For some women, changing to a less demanding program at first may help prepare for the next step. This applies especially to women who have not worked or gone to school for a long time.

WHAT DO YOUR DOCTOR AND TREATMENT TEAM ADVISE?

The expertise and experience of your team can help you assess your readiness to tackle something harder.

HOW FLEXIBLE IS YOUR SCHOOL OR WORK-PLACE?

Women often resume activities part time after a psychotic episode. Will your school or employer understand this and help you arrange it? Will they be flexible in other ways (e.g., your work duties or school assignments)? Do you need your doctor or other care provider to advocate for you? Should you consider a different setting that better suits your needs at this time?

HOW ARE YOUR FINANCES?

Do you have an income or any savings? Are you eligible for financial aid, such as sick benefits, student loans or social assistance?

Other ways to stay well

Keeping appointments with your treatment team and taking medications as prescribed are critical. Discuss any concerns about medications or other aspects of treatment with your doctor or health care worker right away. That way, problems can be addressed. Simply dropping out of treatment or stopping medication without medical advice is very risky, and may lead to a recurrence of psychotic symptoms.

After a psychotic episode, everyone hopes it will never happen again. This is especially true after a first episode. It is important to stay optimistic about the future—but also to be realistic. Having a healthy lifestyle and following treatment advice will give you the best chance of staying well.

If symptoms return, they are best dealt with early. Learn the warning signs of an episode of illness. Discuss these signs with your doctor, counsellor, family members or close friends. Deciding in advance what to do if symptoms reappear helps to avoid a crisis. Some families write down their plan and the phone numbers of people they may need to contact in case of emergency.

5 Family concerns

Feeling strong emotions

Family members may experience many strong emotions, including anxiety, anger, denial, sadness and guilt. All these emotions cause stress, and families all react to stress in different ways.

Communicating

Families dealing with psychosis can find communication frustrating and strained. Kim Mueser and Susan Gingerich (1994) suggest excellent ways to help families communicate after psychosis begins.

These include the following:
- Get to the point. Be clear about what you want to say.
- Express your feelings directly. Use "I" statements. For example, you could say, "I get angry when you do this," rather than "Don't do this!"
- Use praise rather than criticism. For example, you could say, "You got up half an hour earlier today than yesterday. That's wonderful," rather than "You're always getting up late."
- Make positive and explicit requests. For example, you could say,

"Please go to the store before 10 o'clock and buy a quart of milk," rather than "We need milk."
· Check what the other person thinks. Rather than guessing what your relative is thinking or feeling, listen carefully to what the person says. Ask questions when something is unclear. Check whether you correctly understood what you heard.

Working together

You and your family must face some key tasks:
· Find a way to accept that you have had an episode of psychosis and are vulnerable to more episodes.
· Come to terms with the fact that you will likely need medications for a period of time, and possibly indefinitely.
· Become better able to manage your illness. This involves learning everything that you can about your illness and how to stay well. Using this information will help you make healthy choices. This, in turn, will help you control your illness.

Once the psychosis is stabilized, you and your family members will need to work hard to restore balance to your lives. It will help to set some short-, medium- and long-term goals.

6 Planning for the future

Partners

Having a psychotic illness can greatly affect a woman's self-esteem. You may worry that people close to you, including your partner, will reject or leave you. It helps to discuss such feelings with a trusted friend, family member or counsellor.

Sometimes a partner can have fears about the illness that are unfounded. He or she may be able to overcome these fears by getting informed and talking about concerns with a health care professional.

At times, you may not feel good about yourself, and may be lonely. If so, you may be tempted to become intimate with someone you would not normally choose. It is very important not to act impulsively or put yourself at risk. Often, talking to a trusted friend or counsellor about feeling lonely can lead to better solutions.

Children

Some women choose to have children, and some choose not to have children. Typically, women with psychosis have the following questions:

· Should I have a child if I am single?
· Will my child inherit my illness?
· Will I be able to take care of my child?
· Will having a child make me sick again?

What to consider when thinking about having a child

YOUR HEALTH

· Do you have any symptoms that affect your daily activities or relationships?
· How high is your energy level? Do you concentrate well?
· Do your medications make you drowsy?
· Have you had any recent stresses? How well did you cope?
· Have you recently had a relapse and found that you were less able to look after yourself or do normal routines? Who looked after things during this time?
· Is anyone concerned about your ability to look after yourself?
· Are your doctor and health care providers concerned about your ability to care for a baby?

YOUR PARTNER

· How is your partner's health?
· How well does your partner cope with stress?
· How well does your partner understand your illness and its treatment?
· How much is your partner able to help you when you are ill?
· What are your partner's views on having children?
· Is your relationship with your partner likely to continue?
· Do you expect to be a single parent?

YOUR LIVING SITUATION AND FINANCES

· Are you living in a place that would suit a baby (e.g., safe spaces to play, a separate bedroom)? Where you live will affect how well you can look after your child. Subsidized apartments for families may be available.
· Would you have enough money to provide adequately for a baby? To buy food, clothes, toys, other basics?

SUPPORTS

· Do you have family members or friends who could help you with child care? Give financial help if needed?
· If you did have a relapse and needed to be in hospital, who would care for your child?
· If no one could help and child welfare had to take your child into care, how would you feel?
· Would you allow a worker to come to your home and help you care for your child if this was needed?
· Would you be able to attend parenting classes or groups to learn new skills?

YOUR CHILD

· How would you cope if your child developed a mental illness or had learning or behaviour problems, and was harder to manage than average?
· Would you be willing and able to get help for your child if she or he had any special needs?

Talk openly with your partner, other family members, your doctor and other members of your health care team. Note the issues that concern everyone. Then brainstorm about how to address these issues. Research what else you will need to know and how you might find this information. Being well-informed can help a woman and her partner decide whether or not to have a child. It's useful to know about genetic risks, taking medication when pregnant, childbirth and child care.

Will my child inherit my illness?

No one knows exactly how hereditary factors for psychotic illnesses are transmitted. The mental health of both parents contributes to the child's risk.

Schizophrenia is thought to be inherited, but not in a straightforward way. If one parent has schizophrenia, a child has about a one in 10 (10%) chance of inheriting the illness. This is about 10 times more than if the parent did not have schizophrenia. If both parents have schizophrenia, the chances of having a child with the illness are about one in two (50%). Factors such as infection, vitamin deficiency, poor nutrition or substance abuse during pregnancy may increase the risk. Trauma during delivery may also play a role.

Will the authorities take my baby away?

Caring for an infant challenges any woman. You will face extra challenges if you have had psychotic symptoms in the past. You may feel sedated, which is a common side-effect of medication. Or psychotic symptoms may get worse after your baby is born. The chances of being unable to care properly for your baby, and maybe for yourself, are relatively high. In cases like this, a child welfare agency needs to be involved. This is in the best interests of the child and also lessens your responsibility and burden.

You may worry that a child welfare agency will take your child away if they see you struggling. The job of child welfare workers is to ensure the safety and well-being of children. Their goal is not to break up families. Sticking to treatment and working with your treatment team and child welfare worker will increase the chances of your child remaining with you or being returned to you as soon as you are able to cope.

Some infants of parents with a psychotic illness develop slowly. They may be harder to care for than other infants. Having extra help in these cases is important. Your doctor and treatment team can help you arrange this. Public health services offer parenting support. So do many community centres.

7 Finding help

After a psychotic episode, you may want to forget about having
been ill and to stop treatment. It is important, though, to continue
to attend follow-up appointments. This will be a critical time for
you to decide on the next steps in your life. Working with a doctor
and other health care providers will help you address any problems
that arise, and will help you plan to reach your goals. The doctor
who treated your psychotic episode will arrange for you to see a
doctor as an outpatient. A case manager or counsellor may also be
arranged. You may wish to explore other resources, too. Below are
some ideas about where to look for extra help.

A second opinion

At some point in your treatment, you may want a second opinion
on a specific issue, such as your medication or whether to become
pregnant. Most large cities have a hospital-based psychiatric
program linked to a university. These programs are usually doing
research, and have up-to-date information on issues such as new
drugs, genetics and women's mental health. Your doctor can arrange
for you to consult with an expert.

The Canadian Mental Health Association also lists psychiatrists
who specialize in various illnesses. As well, you can contact self-

help organizations, such as the Mood Disorders Association or the Schizophrenia Society. They can suggest experts in the field.

Case management and counselling

Working with a case manager or counsellor who collaborates with a family doctor or psychiatrist can be very helpful. This person will help you plan how to get back to work or school. The counsellor will ensure that you have enough support. A case manager can also work with you and your family members to reduce stress and improve your coping skills.

If you don't have a case manager, ask your doctor to refer you to one. Most hospital programs for outpatients have mental health teams. These teams consist of social workers, nurses, occupational therapists and psychologists, as well as doctors. Community health centres also often have a team of mental health care providers. Organizations offering community care may have services you could benefit from, too. If you are a student, your school will likely have counselling services. Some schools offer specialized services for students with mental health issues. Others may refer you to someone who is able to help you.

Self-help

Organizations such as the Schizophrenia Society and the Mood Disorders Association offer a variety of services, including information meetings with guest speakers, support groups and newsletters. These organizations also advocate for better services and laws. Some hospitals offer self-help groups.

Specialized groups or counsellors

Specialized groups or counsellors address issues such as assertiveness, body image, relationships and trauma, and parenting. Many community-based women's centres offer these services. So do local mental health associations, libraries and mental health clinics.

Alcohol and other drug treatment

Some hospitals and community agencies now offer programs for concurrent disorders. People with concurrent disorders have both a mental illness and a problem with alcohol or other drug use. Check the Internet for alcohol and other drug treatment services in your community.

Pregnancy and medication information

Women who are considering pregnancy or are pregnant may want to consult the Motherisk program at the Hospital for Sick Children in Toronto (tel.: 416 813-6780; website: www.motherisk.org). Motherisk advises pregnant women and health professionals about the possible risks to the fetus. Risks exist when the fetus is exposed to drugs, chemicals, infection or radiation.

Parenting supports

Parents of infants and small children may want one-to-one support and/or to join parenting groups. Public health departments and some community centres and hospitals offer these supports. Most services are free. When a child is at risk, a child welfare agency becomes involved to support the parents, the child and other family members.

A final word

A psychotic illness can dramatically affect a woman and her family. Most women, however, learn to move ahead in life. Here's what you can do:

- Find a doctor and case manager or counsellor you feel you can work with.
- Learn about your illness so you can make informed decisions.
- Work with your health care providers to plan your treatment and recovery.
- Discuss any concerns with your health care providers. That way, you can work together to find solutions.
- Learn how to recognize when the psychosis is coming back. Knowing the signs will help you to act fast.
- Live a balanced life. Take care of your illness. Look after your physical and emotional well-being.
- Find supports and resources you feel will help. Ask for a second opinion if you feel stuck or want someone else's perspective.
- Remember that the solutions that work best for men (the ones in the textbooks) may not work best for women. Make sure your care provider is aware of this.
- Finally, be hopeful. Research is helping to uncover better treatments. Stigma about mental illness is lessening. Life is getting better for people with psychosis.

Related CAMH publications

Baker, S. & Martens, L. (2010). *Promoting Recovery from First Episode Psychosis: A Guide for Families*. Toronto: Centre for Addiction and Mental Health.

Bartha, C., Parker, C., Thomson, C. & Kitchen, K. (2013). *Depression: An Information Guide* (rev. ed.). Toronto: Centre for Addiction and Mental Health.

Bromley, S., Choi, M. & Faruqui, S. (2015). *First Episode Psychosis: A Guide for People with Psychosis and Their Families* (rev. ed.). Toronto: Centre for Addiction and Mental Health.

CAMH Bipolar Clinic Staff. (2013). *Bipolar Disorder: An Information Guide* (rev. ed.). Toronto: Centre for Addiction and Mental Health.

Haskell, L. (2004). *Women, Abuse and Trauma Therapy: An Information Guide for Women and Their Families*. Toronto: Centre for Addiction and Mental Health.

Paterson, J., Butterill, D., Tindall, C., Clodman, D. & Collins, A. (1999). *Schizophrenia: A Guide for People with Schizophrenia and Their Families*. Toronto: Centre for Addiction and Mental Health.

Understanding Psychiatric Medications: Antipsychotics [Pamphlet]. (2012). Toronto: Centre for Addiction and Mental Health.

When a Parent Has Experienced Psychosis . . . What Kids Want to Know [Pamphlet]. (2005). Toronto: Centre for Addiction and Mental Health.

Other guides in this series

Addiction

Anxiety Disorders

Bipolar Disorder

Borderline Personality Disorder

Cognitive-Behavioural Therapy

Concurrent Disorders

Concurrent Substance Use and Mental Health Disorders

Depression

Dual Diagnosis

First Episode Psychosis

The Forensic Mental Health System in Ontario

Obsessive-Compulsive Disorder

Schizophrenia

Women, Abuse and Trauma Therapy